Amine Bahloul
Amine Matari

ECMO: monocentric experiment

Amine Bahloul
Amine Matari

ECMO: monocentric experiment

Observational study on 19 patients.

ScienciaScripts

Imprint

Any brand names and product names mentioned in this book are subject to trademark, brand or patent protection and are trademarks or registered trademarks of their respective holders. The use of brand names, product names, common names, trade names, product descriptions etc. even without a particular marking in this work is in no way to be construed to mean that such names may be regarded as unrestricted in respect of trademark and brand protection legislation and could thus be used by anyone.

Cover image: www.ingimage.com

This book is a translation from the original published under ISBN 978-620-2-54461-0.

Publisher:
Sciencia Scripts
is a trademark of
International Book Market Service Ltd., member of OmniScriptum Publishing Group
17 Meldrum Street, Beau Bassin 71504, Mauritius
Printed at: see last page
ISBN: 978-620-3-17643-8

ECMO: Monocentric experiment: Observational study on 19 patients.

Amine BAHLOUL, Amine MATARI

Colmar Hospital Center

INTRODUCTION

Cardiorespiratory mechanical assistance is most often used intraoperatively to facilitate cardiac surgery (principle of extracorporeal circulation). However, in certain situations, cardiopulmonary assistance operating according to this principle can be used for a longer period of time in a resuscitation unit.

Initially, ECMO was a respiratory assistance technique using a membrane gas exchanger, then by extension ECMO became a respiratory and cardiorespiratory assistance technique. Extended cardiopulmonary *support has* several names: *extracorporeal membrane oxygenation (ECMO)*, extracorporeal *life support* (ECLS), extracorporeal *respiratory support* (AREC), extracorporeal *lung support* (ECLA), extracorporeal *CO2 removal* (ECCO2R).

The ECMO circuit is a simplified CEC circuit. It includes: a venous discharge cannula that drains the blood outside to a pump, this pump returns the blood to a membrane oxygenator and possibly a heater, an arterial or venous injection cannula of the oxygenated blood.

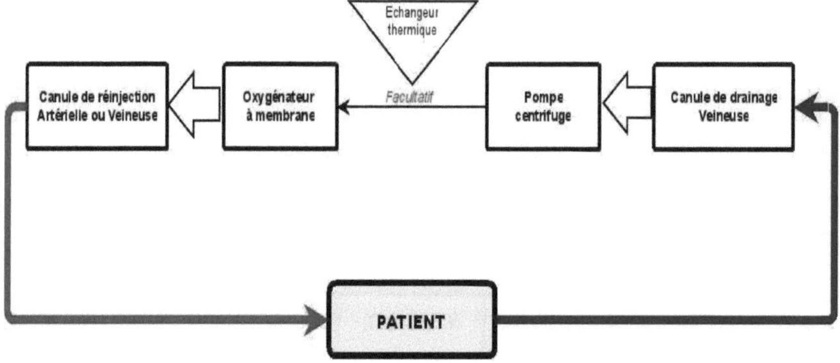

Currently the electric pumps used are essentially non-occlusive centrifugal type, they work according to the vortex effect: rotating rotor that generates the flow and the flow rate.

The flow rate depends not only on the rotation speed but also on the inlet-outlet pressures and the size of the cannulas. The delivered flow rate is continuous and is between 4 and 5 l/min. Flow rate variations are measured by electromagnetic flowmeter and reflect upstream or downstream pressure variations.

The oxygenator reproduces the function of the alveolo-capillary membrane, it therefore comprises a polymethylpentene hollow fiber membrane with a lifetime of approximately 3 weeks. It is connected to a gas mixer (FiO2 and flow rate adjustment). In the oxygenator, the blood is enriched with oxygen (O2), while carbon dioxide (CO2) is removed. Oxygenation depends on the pump flow rate. CO2 removal is independent of blood flow and membrane thickness, but depends on the diffusion gradient, gas flow, membrane surface area, and vacuum at the outlet of the gas circuit [23].

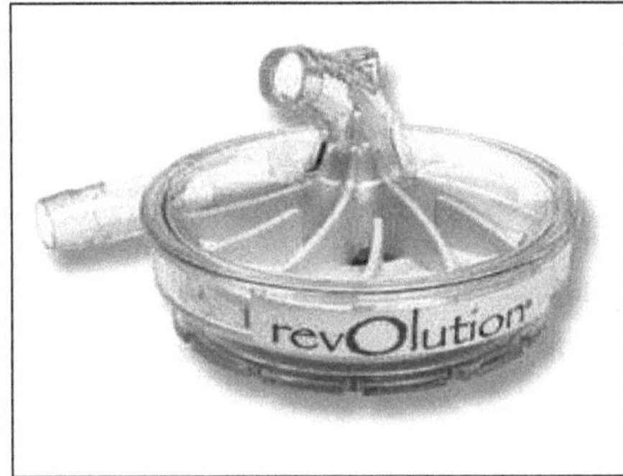

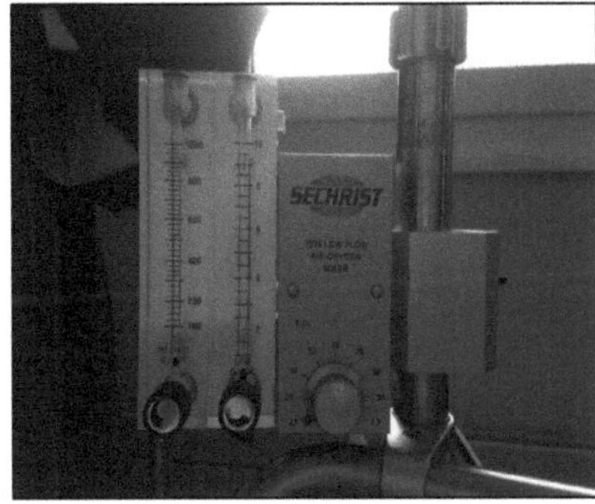

There are two types of ECMO: veno-arterial (VA) and venovenous (VV). During VV ECMO, blood is extracted from the vena cava or right atrium and then re-injected into the right atrium. VV ECMO therefore only provides respiratory assistance, the hemodynamics are assumed to be preserved. For VV ECMO, blood is drawn from the right atrium and re-injected into the arterial system bypassing the heart and lungs, thus providing both respiratory and hemodynamic support. However, the additional benefit of hemodynamic support is offset by additional risks discussed below.

TECHNICAL MODALITIES

1/ Implantation: Once the ECMO indication is established, intravenous heparin anticoagulation is started and the cannulas are inserted, then the pump is switched on as soon as the cannulas are connected to the ECMO circuit.

<u>i) Cannulation:</u> Cannulae are usually placed percutaneously (Seldinger technique). They have a profiled end and a thin, strong wall supported by a metal coil that prevents twisting or bending. The largest possible diameter should be used, especially for the venous cannula (greater flow constraints). For an adult weighing more than 60 kg: arterial cannula between 15 and 19F and venous cannula between 23 and 27F. In our center the cannulas used are: Edwards femoral venous cannula FemTrak™, Medtronic Bio-Medicus® femoral arterial cannula.

For VV ECMO, venous cannulas are generally placed in the right common femoral vein (for drainage) and the right internal jugular vein (for reinjection). The tip of the femoral cannula should be held near the junction of the inferior vena cava and the right atrium, while the tip of the internal jugular cannula should be held near the junction of the superior vena cava and the right atrium. There is also a dual-current cannula wide enough to support 4 to 5 l/min blood flow [24], which is the cannula preferentially used in our center, from the MAQUET Avalon Elite® brand. It is available in a variety of diameters, 31

French being the largest and most suitable for adult men. The drainage and infusion ports have been designed to minimize recirculation. Control of the correct positioning of the venous cannula is imperative, ideally by echocardiography, if not by radiography.

For VA ECMO, femoral access is preferred for the arterial approach because insertion is relatively easy. The main disadvantage of femoral access is

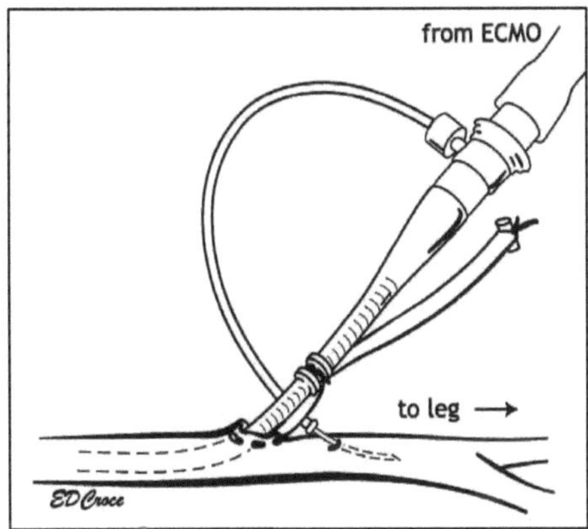

the induced ischemia of the homolateral lower limb. The risk of ischemia can be reduced by inserting an additional distal arterial cannula into the superficial femoral artery to redirect some of the reinjected blood in order to "reperfuse" the lower limb. Alternatively, a cannula may be inserted into the posterior tibial artery to allow retrograde reperfusion [25]. Sometimes the femoral approach is inappropriate for arterial cannulation in the context of VA ECMO (e.g. severe arteriopathy or a history of femoral bypass surgery). In such circumstances, the common carotid artery or right subclavian may be used. There is a risk of massive cerebral infarction when the common carotid artery is used (5-10%). The use of the subclavian artery has the advantage of allowing patients to mobilize [26].

For ECMOs implanted postoperatively in cardiac surgery, the cannulas used for extracorporeal circulation can be transferred to the ECMO circuit for drainage of blood from the right atrium and re-injection into the ascending aorta. The term central ECMO is then used.

ii) Optimization and adjustment: After cannulation, the ECMO circuit is switched on and the pump flow is increased until the hemodynamic and respiratory parameters are satisfactory. The initial objectives are:
- Arterial oxyhemoglobin saturation (SaO2) > 90% for ECMO VA, or > 75% for ECMO VV.
- Venous oxyhemoglobin saturation (SvO2) 70-80% for ECMO VA, measured on the venous line. -
Sufficient tissue perfusion, as determined by blood pressure, SvO2, and lactate level.

2/ Monitoring: Once the initial respiratory and hemodynamic objectives have been reached, the pump flow is maintained. Reassessment and frequent adjustments are facilitated by continuous venous oximetry (SvO2) measured directly on the blood in the venous circuit of the ECMO. When SvO2 is below target, one or more of the following may be increased: flow rate, intravascular volume or hemoglobin concentration (transfusion in case of anemia < 7 g/dl). Decreasing systemic oxygen uptake by reducing temperature may also be helpful.

Anticoagulation is maintained during ECMO by continuous infusion of unfractionated heparin, maintaining an APTT between 180 and 210 seconds or heparinemia between 0.3 and 0.5 IU/ml (standard heparin dose of 50 IU/kg and 100 IU/kg in the absence of a heparin circuit). The APTT target is decreased in case of bleeding.

Thrombocytopenia is common as a result of continuous consumption through platelet activation during extracorporeal exposure. Platelet levels should be maintained above 100,000/microlitre, which may require platelet transfusion.

Ventilation settings are optimized during ECMO to avoid baro or volo trauma (i.e. ventilation-induced lung injury) and oxygen toxicity. Plateau pressure should be maintained < 20 cm H2O with PEEP: 5-10 cm H2O, respiratory rate between 10 and 20 per minute and FiO2 < 50%. The reduction in ventilatory assistance is generally accompanied by an increase in venous return, which improves cardiac output.

An early tracheotomy may be necessary to reduce dead space and improve patient comfort. Patients generally require mild sedation during ECMO, although it is preferable to keep them awake, extubated and breathing spontaneously.

<u>Special Considerations:</u> Each type of ECMO must be taken into account in management.

-Pump Flow: During a VV ECMO, a maximum flow rate is desired to optimize oxygen delivery. However, the flow rate used during VA ECMO should be high enough to provide adequate infusion pressure and venous oxyhemoglobin (SvO2) saturation, but not too high to ensure sufficient preload to maintain left ventricular flow. Any decrease in flow rate corresponds to a decrease in pump filling (hypovolemia, twisting or folding of the venous line, pneumothorax or pericardial effusion interfering with filling), and results in significant fluttering of the venous and arterial lines. Conversely, any increase in flow corresponds to an increase in resistance to ejection (vascular resistance, obstacle on the arterial line).

-Diuresis: Since most patients are in volume overload at the time ECMO is initiated, sufficient diuresis is required once the patient is stable. Ultrafiltration may be added to the ECMO circuit if diuresis is insufficient.

-Cardiac Output Monitoring: Left ventricular output should be carefully monitored during a VA ECMO because of the risk of a drop in cardiac output and an increase in VGDT. This drop in output is usually multifactorial, including underlying left ventricular dysfunction and VG distention related to anterograde flow from the VD and continuous retrograde flow of ECMO in the aorta that increases VG afterload and can lead to irreversible subendocardial ischemia (decreasing the chance of VG recovery) and major hydrostatic pulmonary edema. Left ventricular output can be closely monitored by monitoring BP on an arterial (radial) line and by frequent echocardiography.

3/ Weaning from ECMO: For patients with respiratory failure, radiographic improvement, lung compliance and SaO2 indicate that the patient is ready to be weaned from ECMO. For patients with heart failure, improvement in aortic pulsatility (bloody blood pressure), decreased catecholamine doses, and increased cardiac output on echocardiography correlate with improved VG function and suggest consideration of ECMO withdrawal.

One or more temporary ECMO discontinuation trials should be performed before permanent withdrawal:

- ECMO VV: the tests are performed by stopping the ventilation of the membrane. The extracorporeal blood flow and gas exchanges are progressively reduced to 1 l/min and FiO2 to 21%. Patients are observed for several hours, ventilator parameters necessary to maintain adequate oxygenation and ventilation outside ECMO are determined. Weaning is possible if PaO2 > 60% with FiO2 on the ventilator < 60% and plateau pressure < 30 cmH2O without acute pulmonary heart on echocardiography.

- VA ECMO: the tests require a progressive reduction of the pump flow rate to a minimum flow rate of 1 l/min and then a simultaneous temporary clamping of the two drainage and reinjection lines, while allowing the ECMO circuit to operate through a bridge between the arterial and venous branches, thus avoiding thrombosis due to stagnation within the ECMO circuit. In addition, the arterial and venous lines should be flushed continuously with heparinized saline or intermittently with heparinized blood through the circuit. Withdrawal trials for VA ECMO are generally of shorter duration than for VV ECMO because of the higher risk of thrombus formation. Two echocardiographic parameters predict successful weaning: subaortic ITV $\geq$ 12 cm and lateral mitral ring systolic velocity Sa in DTI $\geq$ 5.8 cm/s.

Once the decision to stop ECMO is made, the cannulas are removed. Hemostasis is achieved by compression of the puncture site. For the arterial puncture site, at least 30 minutes of compression are required. Low doses of Protamine may be administered to reverse the effect of heparin and facilitate hemostasis.

METHODOLOGY

This is a descriptive and qualitative retrospective study with comparison to recent data in the literature. It involved the analysis of the files of patients who have benefited from the implantation of ECMO-type cardiorespiratory assistance. This study covered a period of approximately two years, from June [1,] 2012 to February 13, 2014.

This work was carried out at the Pasteur Hospital in COLMAR. It is a general hospital with a capacity of 748 beds with three Intensive Care Units: Medical Intensive Care Unit of 12 beds, Surgical Intensive Care Unit with general orientation of 12 beds and Surgical Intensive Care Unit with Trauma orientation of 12 beds as well. The Strasbourg University Hospital is considered as the reference center in Cardiac

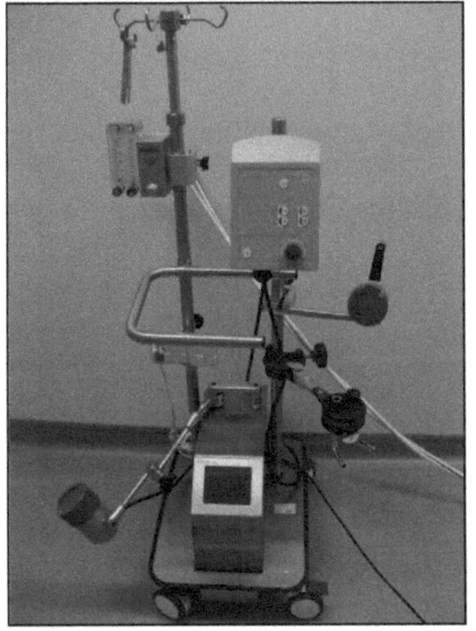

Surgery and is about 70 km away (one hour drive by ambulance).

An ECMO (SORIN Revolution pump model) was acquired at the beginning of 2012 and has been operational since June 2012 after dedicated training of the medical and paramedical staff of the interventional cardiology team and the various intensive care units. Implantation is mainly done percutaneously and is performed by the cardiology team composed of two hemodynamic cardiologists who travel to the different departments if necessary.

Inclusion Criteria: All patients who have benefited from ECMO implantation regardless of the indication.

Exclusion criteria: None as this is a retrospective study.

Data collection: A data collection sheet was used to collect the relevant information. It was compiled on the basis of a literature review. The variables analyzed were : age, sex, notable history, type of ECMO (VV/VA), indication of implantation, biological data including gasometry with PH and Lactates, presence of hepatic or renal dysfunction, echocardiographic parameters with global systolic function (GSF), the presence or not of a significant valvulopathy (aortic insufficiency), the time to implantation and the total duration of ECMO, the need for CPIA (intra aortic balloon counterpulsation), the treatments administered (catecholamines). Finally, the evolutionary data, essentially long-term survival (> 6 months with discharge) and possible complications were noted.

RESULTS

During the study period 19 patients were admitted to CCH and required ECMO.

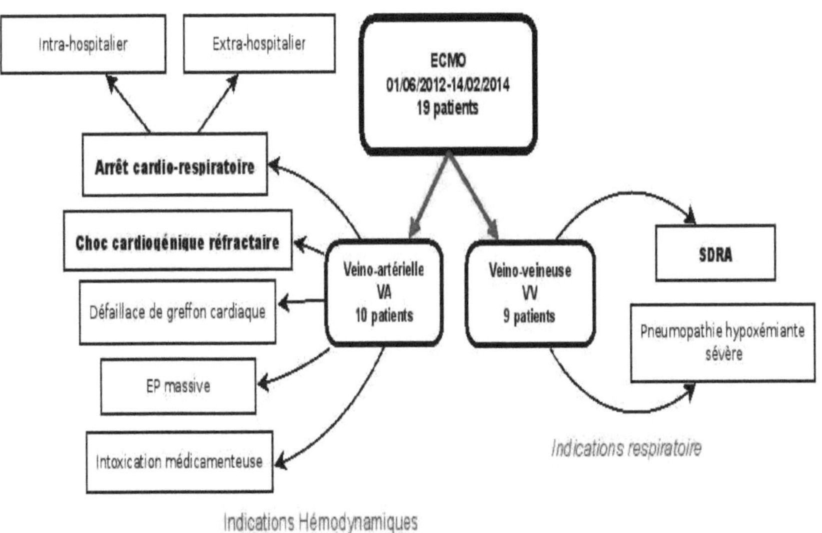

The necessary parameters are missing or incorrect.

Of the 19 patients included, 12 are women (63.15%) and 7 are men (36.85%). The average age is 47.5 years, with the youngest patient at 17 years and the oldest at 76 years.

Among the noteworthy histories are two cardiac transplant patients or 10.5% (congenital cyanogenic heart disease and primary CMD); one patient with biopsy-confirmed exclusively cardiac amyloidosis (5.26%) and another with severe hypertrophic cardiomyopathy (HCM) (5.26%).

Of the 19 patients, nine venovenous or VV ECMOs were implanted (47.37%) and 10 veno-arterial or VA ECMOs (52.63%). Among the VA ECMOs, only two (10.5%) required surgical access (due to morbid obesity). These devices were mostly implanted directly at the patient's bedside in the various intensive care units (13 patients or 68.38%), five times in the catheterization room (5 patients or 26.3%) and only once in the operating room (5.26%).

Table 1lists the type of ECMO implanted and the location of implantation

Location	Type VV	Type VA
Medical Resuscitation	2	4
Surgical resuscitation 2	4	0
Surgical resuscitation 3	3	0
Catheterization room	0	5
Operating room	0	1

The indications for implantation can be roughly divided into respiratory and hemodynamic indications. For respiratory indications, eight patients

(42.1%) benefit from ECMO for Acute Respiratory Distress Syndrome or ARDS: one secondary to a post-traumatic fat embolism (5.26%), one complicating a Legionella septic shock (5.26%), one on an oeso-bronchial fistula complicated by Klebsiella and Candida pneumopathy (5.26%), one post-inhalation chemical ARDS (5.26%), one secondary to drowning (5.26%), two complicating a pneumonectomy (10.5%) and one complicating a chest trauma with pulmonary contusion secondary to a traffic accident (5.26%). There was also a bilateral nosocomial Klebsiella pneumopathy in the aftermath of a head injury (5.26%). The nine previous patients (47.37%) benefited from venovenous ECMO. The remaining ten patients were implanted with veno-arterial ECMO for a hemodynamic indication. Most of them (6, 31.58%) had a cardiorespiratory arrest, including two that occurred out of hospital (10.5%): a rupture of the aorta (post-mortem diagnosis) and acute cardiac graft dysfunction; the other 4 were intra-hospital (21.05%): one patient with isolated cardiac amyloidosis that occurred during endomyocardial biopsy (5.26%), a heart transplant failure dating back 12 years (5.26%), an intraoperative RCA of a nephrectomy with renal vein thrombus that certainly resulted in a pulmonary embolism (5.26%), an RCA at the acute stage of a progressive anterior myocardial infarction managed out of time (5.26%). Two patients presented a cardiogenic shock (10.5%): one on polyintoxic drugs (Nifedipine, antidepressants...) and the other complicating a hypertrophic cardiomyopathy (HCM). Two other patients (10.5%) were victims of a proven massive pulmonary embolism (one by CT scan and the other

directly to angiography) refractory with failure of thrombolysis.

Table 2Main implantation indications with the type of device chosen

Indication	Number	%	Type ECMO
Cardiorespiratory arrest	6	31.58	VA
Refractory cardiogenic shock	2	10.5	VA
Acute Infarction	1	5.26	VA
Graft failure	2	10.5	VA
ARDS	8	42.1	VV
Severe pneumopathy	1	5.26	VV
Massive EP	2	10.5	VA
Drug intoxication	1	5.26	VA

In the veno-arterial ECMO configuration, five patients or 26.3% benefited

from the insertion of an intra-aortic counterpulse balloon (CPIA).

Naturally, all patients required oro-tracheal intubation and catecholamine

infusion to maintain an average blood pressure above 70 mmHg.

Biology was above all the witness of the seriousness of the state of these

patients. All patients with cardiorespiratory arrest, PE or cardiogenic shock were

acidotic with a mean pH of 7.05 ± 0.25 and a mean Lactate level of 17.30 ± 6.70

also indicating low flow and severity of shock. Acute renal failure (mean MDRD GFR 46.6 ml/min) and shock liver with cytolysis and hepatic failure (ASAT 1147 U/L, ALAT 418 U/L, TP 46%) were also noted in these situations. An inflammatory syndrome was observed in 8 patients (42.10%) with median CRP 46 mg/l and mean MDT 12.5 mg/l, this is especially visible in ARDS with bronchopulmonary infection. Cardiomyocyte markers (Troponin I) were increased in all our patients at variable thresholds (mean 1.5 ug/l [0.08-15]) indicating constant myocardial suffering (especially of the right ventricle in respiratory diseases) and in one case (5.26%) related to an acute myocardial infarction with Troponin I at 84 ug/l.

The echocardiography data established the severity of the underlying heart disease and eliminated a possible contraindication (essentially aortic insufficiency, no patients in our series). As expected, for respiratory indications, LVEF was globally conserved (59 ± 6%). On the other hand, in hemodynamic indications, VG systolic dysfunction is almost systematic (average LVEF 46% to be relativized because VG systolic function preserved in PE and HCM).

On a practical level, the lead times before implementation were variable. Quite rapid in the hemodynamic indications of veno-arterial ECMO (mean 7 hours, median 12.5 ± 11.5 hours) and slower in veno-venous ECMO (mean 3.66 days, median 6.5 ± 5.5 days) after consideration with the resuscitators and failure of the conventional therapies used in ARDS (optimization of ventilator settings, ventral decubitus and NO...), these delays may be shorter as experience is gained within the teams. The average duration before weaning was 8 days, with a median of 21 +/- 16 days (up to 37 days!). Several patients had to be transferred to the reference center at the Strasbourg University Hospital, mainly for cardiac surgery (PE embolectomy in 2 cases, mitral plasty of a severe MI by traumatic cord rupture in one patient); otherwise transfer is always considered in the veno-arterial ECMO indication for discussion of circulatory assistance or cardiac transplantation or simply awaiting myocardial recovery in a surgical setting.

Concerning complications (summarized in Table 3), and curiously, no thromboembolic complication is to be deplored or in any case not detected. Finally, as expected, hemorrhagic complications are at the forefront of the table; hemorrhages at the puncture site during or after cannulation in 8 patients (42.10%) with transfusion of red blood cells in all cases, these hemorrhages were controlled in the majority of cases and never led to death; intra-pulmonary hemorrhages, on the other hand, were observed in the veno-arterial ECMO indication in 5 patients (26).31%), pathophysiologically related to a pulmonary alveolar hemorrhagic flood equivalent to PAO in cases of myocardial sideration without any residual contractility as observed in post-cardiac arrest in 3 cases (15.79%), by suture release following a pneumonectomy in one patient (5.26%) and by bleeding from an embolized bronchial artery in another case (5.26%); in addition, cataclysmic hemorrhage (5.26%) on probable rupture of an aortic aneurysm is to be deplored and 2 others on DIC (10.5%).

Poly-visceral failures are noted in 6 patients (31.57%) and systematically lead to the death of these patients. One can also note a severe infectious complication (5.26%) related to Staphylococcus aureus septicaemia with pulmonary abscess on arterial cannula entry portal. Finally, two patients (10.5%) presented a neurological complication that is not directly related to ECMO but rather to the severity of the situations: a post-anoxic coma (5.26%) and regressive resuscitation polyneuropathy (5.26%).

No system-related complications (pump dysfunction) or lower limb ischemia during VA ECMO are observed in our series (systematic insertion of a superficial femoral reperfusion cannula).

Table 3Main complications

Complication	Number	%
Thromboembolic complication	0	0
Neurological impairment	2	10.5
Multi-visceral failure (shock liver, acute renal failure)	6	31.57
Sepsis	5	26.31
Bleeding at the cannulation site	8	42.10
PAO with intra-pulmonary hemorrhage	3	15.79
Limb ischemia	0	0
Complication linked to the device (pump...)	0	0

Finally, of the 19 patients included, there were six survivors at 6 months, all with correct functional status, representing a survival rate of 31.57%. Among these survivors, five had been implanted with venovenous ECMO, i.e. 83% of the survivors and 55.5% of those implanted with VV ECMO, including four for ARDS (one post-traumatic fat embolism, one post-inhalation chemical ARDS, one complicating pulmonary contusion and one following drowning) and one for hypoxemic nosocomial Klebsiella pneumonia. The only survivor (5.26%) of a veno-arterial ECMO was implanted in the context of cardiogenic shock following polyintoxication with drugs (Nifedipine, antidepressants, etc.).

The causes of death are summarized in Table 4, mainly haemorrhage and multisystem failure.

Table 4Causes of death under ECMO

Cause of death	Number	%
Multi-sided failure	6	31.57
Surgical death	1	5.26
Septic shock	1	5.26
Intrapulmonary hemorrhage	4	21.05
Severe hemorrhage (ruptured aortic aneurysm)	1	5.26

DISCUSSION

This retrospective study conducted in a non-university general hospital shows that the need for respiratory or cardio-respiratory assistance is not nil since a total of 19 patients were implanted in less than two years, and that it often has to be decided quickly in patients presenting in an extremely serious or critical condition and therefore difficult to transport in such conditions. The objective of this study is to demonstrate the interest that the availability of this type of device in a peripheral hospital may represent in the management of heavy patients, particularly in terms of survival. Survival of ECMO implanted patients can be classified according to the initial indication: severe acute respiratory or cardiac failure.

In acute respiratory failure, several studies have evaluated the effect of ECMO on mortality [1-11] :

Early observational studies and uncontrolled clinical trials of patients with severe acute respiratory failure have shown survival rates of 50-71% in patients who received ECMO [1-8]. These survival rates were better than the survival rates observed before the advent of this technique.

-A study of 75 patients with severe acute respiratory distress syndrome (ARDS) on H1N1 influenza showed that transfer to an ECMO center was associated with lower intra-hospital mortality (23.7 versus 52.5%) [9]. Eighty-five percent of patients referred to an ECMO center were managed with ECMO, while the remainder improved with conventional ventilation .

-The landmark CESAR (Conventional ventilatory support versus Extracorporeal membrane oxygenation for Severe Acute Respiratory failure trial) randomized 180 patients with ARDS to either a single UK ECMO center or conventional management [10]. The ECMO center group significantly improved disability-free survival at six months compared with conventional management (63 versus 47%). Twenty-five percent of patients referred for ECMO were ultimately not implanted (16 were managed with conventional ventilation and 5 died before transfer to the ECMO center). Note that in this study, severe acute respiratory failure was defined as hypercapnic respiratory acidosis with an arterial pH < 7.20 or a Murray's score greater than 3.0. The Murray score quantifies the severity of respiratory impairment, taking into account the ratio of oxygen partial pressure to inspired oxygen fraction (PaO2/FiO2), positive expiratory pressure (PEP), lung compliance, and chest X-ray. Exclusion criteria included age <18 years or > 65 years, intubation longer than seven days, and contraindications to anticoagulation.

The last two studies described above, conducted in the United Kingdom, show that the use of an ECMO center significantly improves recovery and survival of severe ARDS. In experienced ECMO centers, approximately 25% of patients improve and recover without ECMO, while 75% of patients will require ECMO. Of those who need ECMO, 60-70% will survive. In our study 55.5% of patients implanted with VV ECMO in a respiratory indication survived, which is very close to the data in the literature. This survival rate is likely to improve as more experience is gained.

In heart failure, the results are more mixed and reflect the variety of clinical situations leading to the consideration of this therapy. Observational studies and a few published cases have reported survival rates of 20-43% in patients treated with ECMO VA for cardiac arrest, refractory cardiogenic shock or failed CEC withdrawal after cardiac surgery [12-18]. In two observational studies, ECMO for intra-hospital cardiac arrest was associated with improved survival compared to conventional CPR [19,20].

In the study by Schwartz et al. 46 patients received ECMO (25 for cardiogenic shock and 21 following cardiocirculatory arrest), in this cohort 61% were weaned from ECMO and prolonged survival was 28% and significantly better in the group without initial cardiac arrest [35].

The Pitié-Salpêtrière resuscitation team, which has published extensively in this field, reports the fate of 81 patients who received ECMO for refractory cardiogenic shock. In this study, 42% of the patients came out of resuscitation, 36% were still alive after a median of 11 months while enjoying a good quality of life. Factors associated with death in resuscitation were ECMO implantation under cardiac massage, female sex, and severe hepatic or renal failure [16]. Unfortunately, in our experience, only one patient implanted with veno-arterial ECMO in the context of cardiogenic shock on polyintoxic drugs (Nifedipine, antidepressants...) survived, representing only 10% of patients. The data in the literature effectively highlight the seriousness of these situations and the speed with which hemodynamic assistance must be implemented in these cases before signs of multi-visceral failure appear, and this is why a Mobile Circulatory Assistance Unit (MACU) [16] or the presence of ECMO in general hospitals is so important to improve the morbidity and mortality of these serious cases.

Naturally, the management of these patients can only be conceived afterwards in a university center experienced in the management of such patients and especially near a surgical environment. The poor figures reported in our work are to be correlated with the fact that the majority of our patients were treated for extremely precarious conditions, as six of the ten patients implanted with VA ECMO were in the context of cardiopulmonary arrest, A situation in which poor results are well highlighted in previous studies, which insist that in the event of intra-hospital or a fortiori extra-hospital cardiocirculatory arrest, the implementation of therapeutic ECMO must be discussed on the basis of very strict criteria [38, 34, 20, 13, 39]; the prognosis being clearly worse in case of No-flow >

5 minutes and Low-flow > 100 minutes (or ETCO2 < 10 mmHg), a management

algorithm has been proposed by a French multi-disciplinary group [40].

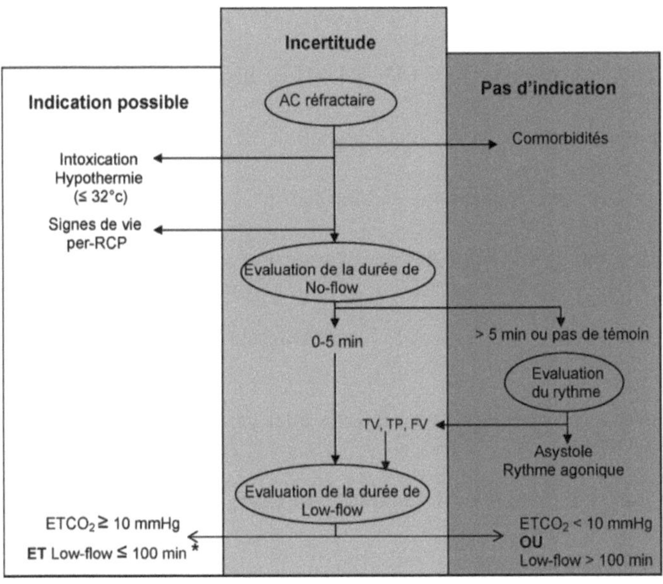

Recommendations concerning the practical indications for ECMO have

been published by the ELSO (Extracorporeal Life Support Organization) [22]

which summarize the clinical situations in which ECMO implantation is

discussed in both respiratory and cardiac failure situations:

-Hypoxemic respiratory failure with PaO2/FiO2 ratio <100 mm Hg despite

optimized ventilator settings including tidal volume, positive expiratory pressure

(PEEP), and I:E ratio despite use of adjunctive therapies such as inhaled NO [

48] and prone decubitus [49, 50].

-Respiratory failure hypercapnia with arterial pH < 7.20

Refractory cardiogenic shock with high recovery potential (myocarditis [43], stress heart disease or drug intoxication with a cardio-toxic substance with a membrane-stabilizing effect [38, 44, 45]), myocardial infarction [42], acute decompensation of CMD, acute rejection of a heart transplant [46], more exceptionally severe pulmonary embolism [47]; in some cases as a bridge to a heart transplant or the implantation of a definitive ventricular assistance.

-Refractory cardiac arrest, mostly intra-hospital [44, 34, 20, 13, 39].

-Difficulties in withdrawal from Bypass after cardiac surgery [41].

-Polytrauma: hemodynamic support in case of myocardial contusion and ventilatory support in case of pulmonary contusion

ECMO may therefore be a last resort solution to improve prognosis in particularly critical situations at the cost of certain morbidity. It is indeed a heavy device requiring experience and logistics within multidisciplinary teams experienced in the management of such devices which, in return for a proven service, are burdened with frequent complications, sometimes serious or even fatal.

In the literature, hemorrhages concern 30 to 40% of patients on ECMO, and are potentially fatal. We have listed 8 of them in our series, i.e. 42.10%. They are favored by heparin infusion and thrombocytopenia. Surgical implantation of the cannulas, maintenance of a platelet count above 100,000/mm3, and maintenance of a target APTT ratio reduce the risk of bleeding. Intervention is necessary when major bleeding occurs. Local bleeding at the cannulation site often requires surgical repositioning. Internal bleeding (abdomen, pleura) requires surgical exploration for hemostasis and drainage. Antifibrinolytic procoagulant therapy with a plasminogen activation inhibitor (aminocaproic acid, tranexamic acid) may be used or interruption of heparin infusion for several hours, but these actions may increase the risk of circuit thrombosis [27-29]. A few teams have tried infusions of activated factor VII (Novoseven®) with mixed results, the latter possibility being reserved for extreme cases when all other options have failed [30,31]. The target APTT is generally reduced in the event of hemorrhage. A target TCA at 170-190 seconds instead of 210-230 seconds seems reasonable.

Systemic embolism due to thrombus formation in the extracorporeal circuit is a rare complication with a very poor prognosis. Its impact is greater with VA ECMO since it occurs in the systemic circulation. The occurrence of thrombi increases with the duration of ECMO. Heparin infusion with a good APTT target and regular checking of the ECMO circuit for clotting help prevent this complication. Observation of the ECMO circuit for clots includes routine inspection of all connectors and measurement of the pressure gradient across the oxygenator. An abrupt change in the pressure gradient suggests that a thrombus may have formed. A large moving thrombus requires immediate circuit interruption or replacement. A purged, ready-to-use replacement circuit is usually kept nearby when the target APTT has been reduced due to bleeding because the risk of thrombus formation is greater in this situation. Systematically, consideration should be given to replacing the membrane and circuit after 12 to 15 days of operation. Fortunately, no thrombosis was reported in our study.

Vascular complications related to cannulation such as perforation of a vessel with hemorrhage, arterial dissection, distal ischemia, implantation error (venous cannula in the artery) are possible. These complications are rare (< 5%). Surgical intervention may be necessary.

In cases of proven heparin-induced thrombocytopenia (HIT type 2), the heparin infusion should be replaced by a non-heparin anticoagulant [32]. Argatroban is preferred because of its short half-life and identical APTT target.

One patient (5.26%) in our series presented with Staphylococcus aureus septicemia complicated by pulmonary abscess on call point at the cannula. Infectious complications are observed in 15 to 20% of cases, mainly cellulitis of the peripheral femoral cannula implantation site (mediastinitis in case of central ECMO).

Neurological impairment is considered to be relatively rare in adult ECMO survivors, which our series corroborates since two patients (10.5%) have presented this complication, which is as much the consequence of the initial pathology that motivated the initiation of ECMO, as a direct complication of ECMO: a post-anoxic coma (5.26%) and regressive resuscitation polyneuropathy (5.26%). A prospective cohort study of patients implanted with ECMO for more than 12 hours showed neurological impairment in 42 patients (approximately 50%) [21]. The types of neurological impairment identified were coma of uncertain cause (11 patients), encephalopathy (11 patients), anoxic brain injury (9 patients), hemorrhage (7 patients), brain death (3 patients), and myoclonus (1 patient).

Finally, some complications are specific to VA ECMO and explain the higher morbidity compared to VV ECMO:

- Pulmonary hydrostatic edema and pulmonary hemorrhage, usually fatal, that claimed the lives of three of our patients (15.79%) who suffered cardiorespiratory arrest. Left ventricular output must be rigorously monitored during VA ECMO because of the risk of a drop in cardiac output and an increase in PTDVG. This drop in output is usually multifactorial, including underlying left ventricular dysfunction and VG distention related to anterograde flow from the VD and continuous retrograde flow of ECMO in the aorta increasing VG afterload and possibly leading to irreversible subendocardial ischemia (decreasing the chances of VG recovery) and major hydrostatic pulmonary edema with pulmonary hemorrhage. Left ventricular output can be closely monitored by monitoring BP on an arterial (radial) line and by frequent echocardiography. Some interventions may improve the performance of VG: **i) inotropic** agents (dobutamine) to increase contractility, **ii) intra-aortic counterpulse balloon (CPBIA)** [37] to reduce afterload and facilitate VG ejection, **iii)** immediate VG **decompression** may be essential to avoid pulmonary hemorrhage if VG flow cannot be maintained despite CPBIA and inotropic agents. This can be achieved by percutaneous atrial septotomy, percutaneous insertion of a cannula into the left atrium after trans-septal catheterization, placement of left percutaneous assistance with an Impella® type catheter [36] or surgical thoracotomy, and insertion of a discharge cannula into a pulmonary vein or at the tip of the VG. Finally, conversion to central ECMO (CEC) may be considered.

- Cardiac Thrombosis: Blood stasis may occur with low cardiac output associated with continuous retrograde ECMO blood flow in the ascending aorta, which can lead to thrombosis.

- Coronary or cerebral hypoxia: During VA ECMO, blood that is fully saturated with oxygen tends to preferentially irrigate the lower limbs and intra-abdominal viscera. The blood ejected by the VG, on the other hand, selectively perfuses the heart, brain and upper limbs. As a result, the oxyhemoglobin saturation of blood perfusing the lower extremities and abdominal viscera may be significantly higher than that perfusing the heart, brain and upper extremities. Cardiac and cerebral hypoxia may occur and be unrecognized if oxygen saturation is monitored only on blood drawn from the lower extremities. To avoid this complication, arterial oxyhemoglobin (SaO_2) saturation should be monitored both in the upper limbs (radial gasometry or finger pulse oximetry) and lower limbs (femoral gasometry). Poor arterial oxyhemoglobin (SaO_2) saturation measured in the upper limb can be corrected by infusion of oxygenated blood into the right atrium.

CONCLUSION

The objective of this small retrospective study was to review the literature on ECMO, to compare itself with this data and finally to demonstrate the interest that a general hospital center may have in being able to initiate, monitor and manage this type of therapy with a view to improving mortality, particularly in extreme situations.

In the slightly less than two years that our center has had it, there have been encouraging signs, particularly in the respiratory indications of venovenous ECMO, where slightly more than half of the patients have survived with a satisfactory quality of life, the majority having been cared for locally throughout their hospitalization. On the other hand, efforts still need to be made in the management of heart failure by veno-arterial ECMO. Only one patient probably survived thanks to the good initial indication since she was the only one to present a heart failure with a high recovery potential (intoxication with drugs with a membrane-stabilizing effect). The other patients presented most often cardio-circulatory arrests (6 patients out of 10) often out of hospital, sometimes requiring implantation under external cardiac massage, and died in most cases of multi-visceral failure, cataclysmic hemorrhages on DICD or PAO with pulmonary hemorrhage.

All of these elements should encourage emergency physicians, cardiologists and resuscitators to quickly recognize pathologies likely to evolve early towards refractory cardiogenic shock and asystole in order to consider starting ECMO in the shortest possible time. The interest of ECMO in the management of out-of-hospital cardiac arrest is still subject to debate...

REFERENCES:

1.   Hemmila MR, Rowe SA, Boules TN, et al. Extracorporeal life support for severe acute respiratory distress syndrome in adults. Ann Surg 2004; 240:595.

2.   Peek GJ, Moore HM, Moore N, et al. Extracorporeal membrane oxygenation for adult respiratory failure. Chest 1997; 112:759.

3.   Lewandowski K, Rossaint R, Pappert D, et al. High survival rate in 122 ARDS patients managed according to a clinical algorithm including extracorporeal membrane oxygenation. Intensive Care Med 1997; 23:819.

4.   Ullrich R, Lorber C, Röder G, et al. Controlled airway pressure therapy, nitric oxide inhalation, prone position, and extracorporeal membrane oxygenation (ECMO) as components of an integrated approach to ARDS. Anesthesiology 1999; 91:1577.

5.   Rich PB, Awad SS, Kolla S, et al. An approach to the treatment of severe adult respiratory failure. J Crit Care 1998; 13:26.

6.   Kolla S, Awad SS, Rich PB, et al. Extracorporeal life support for 100 adult patients with severe respiratory failure. Ann Surg 1997; 226:544.

7.   Australia and New Zealand Extracorporeal Membrane Oxygenation (ANZ ECMO) Influenza Investigators, Davies A, Jones D, et al. Extracorporeal Membrane Oxygenation for 2009 Influenza A(H1N1) Acute Respiratory Distress Syndrome. JAMA 2009; 302:1888.

8.   Brogan TV, Thiagarajan RR, Rycus PT, et al. Extracorporeal membrane oxygenation in adults with severe respiratory failure: a multi-center database. Intensive Care Med 2009; 35:2105.

9.   Noah MA, Peek GJ, Finney SJ, et al. Referral to an extracorporeal membrane oxygenation center and mortality among patients with severe 2009 influenza A(H1N1). JAMA 2011; 306:1659.

10.   Peek GJ, Mugford M, Tiruvoipati R, et al. Efficacy and economic assessment of conventional ventilatory support versus extracorporeal membrane oxygenation for severe adult respiratory failure (CESAR): a multicentre randomised controlled trial. Lancet 2009; 374:1351.

11.   Pham T, Combes A, Rozé H, et al. Extracorporeal membrane oxygenation for pandemic influenza A(H1N1)-induced acute respiratory distress syndrome: a cohort study and propensity-matched analysis. Am J Respir Crit Care Med 2013; 187:276.

12.   Younger JG, Schreiner RJ, Swaniker F, et al. Extracorporeal resuscitation of cardiac arrest. Acad Emerg Med 1999; 6:700.

13.   Massetti M, Tasle M, Le Page O, et al. Back from irreversibility: extracorporeal life support for prolonged cardiac arrest. Ann Thorac Surg 2005; 79:178.

14.   Smedira NG, Blackstone EH. Postcardiotomy mechanical support: risk factors and outcomes. Ann Thorac Surg 2001; 71:S60.

15.   Kelly RB, Porter PA, Meier AH, et al. Duration of cardiopulmonary resuscitation before extracorporeal rescue: how long is not long enough? ASAIO J 2005; 51:665.

16.   Combes A, Leprince P, Luyt CE, et al. Outcomes and long-term quality-of-life of patients supported by extracorporeal membrane oxygenation for refractory cardiogenic shock. Crit Care Med 2008; 36:1404.

17.   Pagani FD, Aaronson KD, Swaniker F, Bartlett RH. The use of extracorporeal life support in adult patients with primary cardiac failure as a bridge to implantable left ventricular assist device. Ann Thorac Surg 2001; 71:S77.

18.   Kagawa E, Dote K, Kato M, et al. Should we emergently revascularize occluded coronaries for cardiac arrest?: Rapid-response extracorporeal membrane oxygenation and intra-arrest percutaneous coronary intervention. Circulation . Published online ahead of print, August 16, 2012.

19.   Shin TG, Choi JH, Jo IJ, et al. Extracorporeal cardiopulmonary resuscitation in patients with inhospital cardiac arrest: A comparison with conventional cardiopulmonary resuscitation. Crit Care Med 2011; 39:1.

20.   Chen YS, Lin JW, Yu HY, et al. Cardiopulmonary resuscitation with assisted extracorporeal life-support versus conventional cardiopulmonary resuscitation in adults with in-hospital cardiac arrest: an observational study and propensity analysis. Lancet 2008; 372:554.

21.   Mateen FJ, Muralidharan R, Shinohara RT, et al. Neurological injury in adults treated with extracorporeal membrane oxygenation. Arch Neurol 2011; 68:1543.

22.   ELSO guidelines for ECMO centers (updated March 2014) http://www.elsonet.org/index.php?option=com_phocadownload&view=category &id=4&Itemid=627

23.   Schmidt M, Tachon G, Devilliers C, et al. Blood oxygenation and decarboxylation determinants during venovenous ECMO for respiratory failure in adults. Intensive Care Med 2013; 39:838.

24.   Wang D, Zhou X, Liu X, et al. Wang-Zwische double lumen cannula-toward a percutaneous and ambulatory paracorporeal artificial lung. ASAIO J 2008; 54:606.

25.   Madershahian N, Nagib R, Wippermann J, et al. A simple technique of distal limb perfusion during prolonged femoro-femoral cannulation. J Card Surg 2006; 21:168.

26.   Navia JL, Atik FA, Beyer EA, Ruda Vega P. Extracorporeal membrane oxygenation with right axillary artery perfusion. Ann Thorac Surg 2005; 79:2163.

27.   Wilson JM, Bower LK, Fackler JC, et al. Aminocaproic acid decreases the incidence of intracranial hemorrhage and other hemorrhagic complications of ECMO. J Pediatr Surg 1993; 28:536.

28.   Biswas AK, Lewis L, Sommerauer JF. Aprotinin in the management of life-threatening bleeding during extracorporeal life support. Perfusion 2000; 15:211.

29.   Peek, G, Wittenstein, et al. Management of bleeding during ECLS. In: ECMO in Critical Care, Van Meurs, K, Lally, KP, Peek, G, Zwischenberger, JB (Eds), Extracorporeal life support organization, Ann Arbor 2005.

30.   Bui JD, Despotis GD, Trulock EP, et al. Fatal thrombosis after administration of activated prothrombin complex concentrates in a patient supported by extracorporeal membrane oxygenation who had received activated recombinant factor VII. J Thorac Cardiovasc Surg 2002; 124:852.

31.   Wittenstein B, Ng C, Ravn H, Goldman A. Recombinant factor VII for severe bleeding during extracorporeal membrane oxygenation following open heart surgery. Pediatr Crit Care Med 2005; 6:473.

32.   Cornell T, Wyrick P, Fleming G, et al. A case series describing the use of argatroban in patients on extracorporeal circulation. ASAIO J 2007; 53:460.

33.   Thiele H, Sick P, Boudriot E, et al. Randomized comparison of intra-aortic balloon support with a percutaneous left ventricular assist device in patients with revascularized acute myocardial infarction complicated by cardiogenic shock. Eur Heart J 2005; 26:1276.

34. Chen YS, Yu HY, Huang SC, Lin JW, Chi NH, Wang CH, et al. Extracorporeal membrane oxygenation support can extend the duration of cardiopulmonary resuscitation. Crit Care Med 2008;36:2529-35.

35. Schwarz B, Mair P, Margreiter J, Pomaroli A, Hoermann C, Bonatti J, et al. Experience with percutaneous venoarterial cardiopulmonary bypass for emergency circulatory support. Crit Care Med 2003;31:758-64.

36. Vlasselaers D, Desmet M, Desmet L, Meyns B, Dens J. Ventricu- lar unloading with a miniature axial flow pump in combination with extracorporeal membrane oxygenation. Intensive Care Med 2006;32:329-33.

37. Sauren LD, Reesink KD, Selder JL, Beghi C, van der Veen FH, Maessen JG. The acute effect of intra-aortic balloon counter- pulsation during extracorporeal life support: an experimental study. Artif Organs 2007;31:31-8.

38. Megarbane B, Leprince P, Deye N, Resiere D, Guerrier G, Ret- tab S, et al. Emergency feasibility in medical intensive care unit of extracorporeal life support for refractory cardiac arrest. Intensive Care Med 2007;33:758-64.

39. Chen YS, Chao A, Yu HY, Ko WJ, Wu IH, Chen RJ, et al. Analysis and results of prolonged resuscitation in cardiac arrest patients rescued by extracorporeal membrane oxygenation. J Am Coll Cardiol 2003;41:197-203.

40 Recommendations on the indications for circulatory support in the treatment of refractory cardiac arrest. 2008.

http://www.srlf.org/mediatheque/conferencerecommandations/cardiocirculatoire/indications-de-l-assistance-circulatoire-dans-le-traitement-des-arrets-cardiaques-refractaires.r.phtml

41.   Bakhtiary F, Keller H, Dogan S, Dzemali O, Oezaslan F, Meininger D, et al. Venoarterial extracorporeal membrane oxygenation for treatment of cardiogenic shock: clinical experiences in 45 adult patients. J Thorac Cardiovasc Surg 2008;135:382-8.

42.   Chen JS, Ko WJ, Yu HY, Lai LP, Huang SC, Chi NH, et al. Analysis of the outcome for patients experiencing myocardial infarction and cardiopulmonary resuscitation refractory to conventional therapies necessitating extracorporeal life support rescue. Crit Care Med 2006;34:950-7.

43   Feldman AM, McNamara D. Myocarditis. N Engl J Med 2000;343: 1388-98.

44.   Holzer M, Sterz F, Schoerkhuber W, Behringer W, Doma- novits H, Weinmar D, et al. Successful resuscitation of a verapamil-intoxicated patient with percutaneous cardiopulmo- nary bypass. Crit Care Med 1999;27:2818-23.

45.Goodwin DA, Lally KP, Null Jr DM. Extracorporeal membrane oxygenation support for cardiac dysfunction from tricyclic anti- depressant overdose. Crit Care Med 1993;21:625-7.

46.   Magovern Jr GJ, Simpson KA. Extracorporeal membrane oxy- genation for adult cardiac support: the Allegheny experience. Ann Thorac Surg 1999;68:655-61.

47.   Schwarz B, Mair P, Margreiter J, Pomaroli A, Hoermann C, Bonatti J, et al. Experience with percutaneous venoarterial cardiopulmonary bypass for emergency circulatory support. Crit Care Med 2003;31:758-64.

48.   Adhikari NK, Burns KE, Friedrich JO, Granton JT, Cook DJ, Meade MO. Effect of nitric oxide on oxygenation and morta- lity in acute lung injury: systematic review and meta-analysis. BMJ 2007;334:779.

49.   Mancebo J, Fernandez R, Blanch L, Rialp G, Gordo F, Ferrer M, et al. A multicenter trial of prolonged prone ventilation in severe acute respiratory distress syndrome. Am J Respir Crit Care Med 2006;173:1233-9.

50.   Guerin C, Gaillard S, Lemasson S, Ayzac L, Girard R, Beuret P, et al. Effects of systematic prone positioning in hypoxemic acute respiratory failure: a randomized controlled trial. JAMA 2004;292:2379-87.

TABLE OF CONTENTS

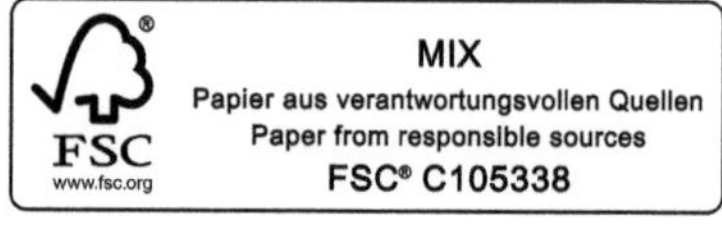
Printed by Books on Demand GmbH, Norderstedt / Germany